2024 Fresh Start

Top 10 Diet Secrets for a Vibrant New Year

Evelyn C. Kohl

Copyright

All rights reserved. No part of this publication may be reproduced, distributed, or transmitted in any form or any means, including photocopying, recording or other electronic or mechanical methods, without the prior written permission of the publisher, except in the case of brief quotations embodied in critical reviews and certain other non-commercial uses permitted by copyright law.

Copyright © (Evelyn C. Kohl), (2024).

About the author

Evelyn C. Kohl is a respected author who is known for adding new and thought-provoking ideas to the body of health and wellness writing. Evelyn is a recognised voice in helping people reach their wellness goals. She has a background in nutritional science and a strong desire to promote healthy lifestyles.

Evelyn's journey began when she studied nutrition and dietetics and did very well. She was motivated by a strong belief that food can change both the body and the mind. Early in her career, she worked closely with people from a wide range of backgrounds to help them understand the basics of nutrition and how the food they eat can affect their health as a whole.

Evelyn is unique because she can take complicated nutritional ideas and turn them into easy-to-understand, useful tips. Her writing is clear and warm, and it connects with readers on a human level. This makes the journey to health and wellness both possible and fun. She is very good at writing material that is not only useful but also interesting and relatable, which is why her fans stick with her.

Her books are often about how to combine science and everyday life. They are full of personal stories that make her advice feel relevant and genuine. She talks about how important balance is and supports a whole-person attitude to health and diet. Evelyn's work often addresses the psychological aspects of eating and health, offering strategies for mindful eating, stress reduction, and developing a positive relationship with food.

Evelyn's impact goes beyond the books she wrote. She is a sought-after speaker and consultant, known for her dynamic workshops and seminars that encourage people to make sustainable lifestyle changes. Her blog and social media platforms are treasure troves of useful tips, healthy recipes, and motivational insights.

In her personal life, Evelyn embodies the beliefs she preaches. She is an avid cook, a yoga lover, and a proponent of sustainable living. Her approach to life is one of balance and harmony, and she finds joy in helping others discover their way to a healthier, happier life.

Through her writing and teaching, Evelyn C. Kohl continues to inspire a new generation of readers to accept a more mindful, healthful approach to living, making her a true luminary in the field of health and wellness literature.

Table of Content

Introduction

Embracing a Healthier 2024: The Importance of Starting Fresh

As we usher in 2024, it presents a unique chance to reset and embrace a healthier lifestyle. The concept of starting fresh is not just a symbolic gesture but a powerful psychological tool that can spur major changes in our lives. The new year is synonymous with new starts, and there's no better time to reevaluate and redefine our health goals.

Starting fresh means leaving behind old habits that don't serve our wellbeing and choosing new, healthier ones. It's about looking at our health holistically, knowing that small, consistent changes can lead to substantial long-term benefits. This fresh start isn't just about diet; it extends to all aspects of health and wellness, including physical exercise, mental health, and emotional well-being.

This approach is particularly important after the challenges and stresses of the past years. Many of us have experienced changes in our habits, perhaps leading to less-than-ideal health choices. A fresh start in 2024 is a chance to leave behind the sedentary habits and stress-eating patterns and move towards a more balanced and healthy lifestyle.

What to Expect from These Top 10 Diet Secrets

1. Holistic Approach to Diet:

These secrets aren't just about losing weight; they're about nurturing your body with the right nutrients, finding a sustainable way of eating, and knowing how food affects not just your body but also your mood and energy levels.

2. Evidence-Based Advice:

Expect recommendations grounded in scientific study. These secrets draw from the latest studies in nutrition and dietetics, ensuring you're getting help that's not only effective but also safe and healthy.

3. **Customizable Strategies**:

Everyone's body and lifestyle are different, and there's no one-size-fits-all method to diet. These secrets provide flexible guidelines that can be changed to suit individual needs, preferences, and goals.

4. **Focus on Plant-Based Foods**:

You'll learn about the benefits of incorporating more plant-based foods into your diet, including how they can reduce the risk of chronic diseases, improve gut health, and support general wellness.

5. **Hydration and its Benefits**:

Hydration is often overlooked in diet talks, but it's a key component of health. These tips will delve into the importance of staying hydrated and how it can improve digestion, skin health, and energy levels.

6. **Mindful Eating Practices**:

Moving away from diets focused on restrictions, these secrets support a more mindful approach to eating. This includes listening to your body's hunger cues, enjoying your food, and knowing the psychological aspects of eating.

7. **Sugar and Processed Foods**:

You'll get practical advice on how to reduce sugar and processed foods in your diet, which is important for reducing the risk of obesity, diabetes, and other health issues.

8. Balancing Macronutrients:

Understand the roles of proteins, carbohydrates, and fats in your food and how to balance them effectively for optimal health.

9. Meal Planning and Preparation:

Learn how to plan and prepare your meals in advance to ensure you're eating healthy, balanced meals throughout the week.

10. Consistency Over Perfection:

Finally, these secrets stress the importance of consistency over perfection. It's about making gradual changes and knowing that occasional indulgences are part of a balanced diet.

In summary, "2024 Fresh Start: Top 10 Diet Secrets for a Vibrant New Year" is more than just a diet plan; it's a complete guide to overhauling your relationship with food and nourishment. By embracing these secrets, you're not just starting on a short-term diet; you're taking the first steps towards a healthier, more vibrant life in the new year and beyond.

Secret #1

Power of Plant-Based Choices

Benefits of Adding More Greens

Nutritional Value:

Greens are dietary forces to be reckoned with, loaded with nutrients, minerals, and fiber, yet low in calories. Leafy greens like spinach, kale, and Swiss chard are rich in iron, calcium, potassium, and magnesium, along with vitamins A, C, E, and K. They also provide a number of phytonutrients – compounds that help protect plants from germs, fungi, bugs, and other threats, and can also benefit human health.

Health Benefits:

Regular eating of greens can lead to numerous health benefits. They're known for their ability to reduce the chance of chronic diseases such as heart disease, diabetes, and certain cancers. The fiber in greens aids in digestion and can help keep a healthy gut microbiome. They also play a crucial role in keeping healthy skin and hair, and can help with weight management due to their low calorie yet high nutrient content.

Mental and Emotional Health:

Recent studies have shown a link between the consumption of greens and mental health. Nutrients found in greens, such as folate, can play a role in lowering depression symptoms. Greens also contain antioxidants that fight reactive stress, which can affect brain health.

Easy Plant-Based Swaps for Everyday Meals

Breakfast Swaps:
- Oatmeal or Smoothie Bowls: Top your oatmeal or smoothie bowls with a handful of spinach or kale. These greens blend well without altering the taste greatly.

- Tofu Scramble: Replace standard scrambled eggs with a tofu scramble. Add turmeric for color and a range of vegetables for a nutritious start to your day.

- Butter to Avocado: Use mashed avocado as a spread on toast instead of butter for a healthy dose of natural fats.

Lunch Swaps:

- Salads: Incorporate a mix of leafy greens like lettuce, arugula, spinach, and kale. These not only add different textures and flavors but also improve your nutrient intake.
- Wraps and Sandwiches: Add veggies like spinach, kale, or lettuce to your wraps and sandwiches. Even an easy addition like this can make a regular sandwich much healthier.

- Chicken or Tuna Salad to Chickpea Salad: Mash chickpeas and mix with vegan mayo, mustard, diced celery, and onions for a plant-based salad sandwich filler.

- Cheese in Sandwiches to Hummus: Spread hummus on sandwiches or wraps for creaminess and flavor, plus extra protein and fiber.

- Cream-Based Soups to Vegetable Broth or Coconut Milk: For creamy soups, use blended cashews, coconut milk, or pureed veggies as a base instead of dairy cream.

Dinner Swaps:

- Stir-Fries: Add greens like bok choy, spinach, or Swiss chard to your stir-fries. They cook quickly and add a fresh, crunchy taste.

- Pasta Dishes: Mix in spinach or kale into your pasta recipes. They wilt down and blend easily into dishes like spaghetti or lasagna.

- Ground Beef to Lentils or Quinoa: In recipes like tacos, spaghetti, or casseroles, use cooked lentils or quinoa as a protein-rich, plant-based substitute.

- Steak or Chicken to Portobello Mushrooms: Grill or roast portobello mushrooms as a meaty, flavorful substitute in burgers or main meals.

- Butter in Cooking to Olive or Avocado Oil: Swap butter for olive oil or avocado oil when sautéing or roasting veggies.

Snack Swaps:
- Green Smoothies: Blend together fruits and a handful of greens like spinach or kale for a quick, nutrient-packed lunch.

- Baked Goods: Add veggies like spinach to your muffins or pancakes. Spinach, in particular, can be easily hidden in baked goods, making it a great way to sneak in extra nutrients.

- Yogurt to Plant-Based Yogurt: Opt for soy, almond, or coconut-based yogurts for a vegan snack or dessert choice.

- Cheese Crackers to Nut-Based Crackers: Choose crackers made from almonds, flaxseeds, or other nuts and seeds for a crunchy, healthy snack.

Beverage Swaps:

- Green Juices: Combine fresh greens with fruits like apples or oranges for a sweet, nutrient-rich drink.

- Herbal drinks: Consider drinks with moringa or matcha, which are both derived from green leaves and are packed with antioxidants.

- Cow's Milk to Nut Milk in Smoothies: Use almond, cashew, or oat milk in your shakes for a creamy texture without dairy.

- Cream in Coffee to Nut Creamers: There are different plant-based creamers available, made from almonds, oats, or coconuts, which are great in coffee or tea.

- Desserts Milk Chocolate to Dark Chocolate: Dark chocolate is often dairy-free and a healthier choice rich in antioxidants.

- Ice Cream to Banana Nice Cream: Blend frozen bananas until creamy for an easy, natural, and dairy-free ice cream alternative.

- Baking with Eggs to Flax or Chia Eggs: Mix 1 tablespoon of ground flaxseed or chia seeds with 3 tablespoons of water to replace one egg in baking recipes.

General Cooking

- Buttermilk to Plant-Based Buttermilk: Mix plant-based milk with a tablespoon of lemon juice or vinegar to replicate buttermilk.

- Honey to Agave or Maple Syrup: Use agave nectar or maple syrup as a natural sweetener instead of honey.

- Gelatin to Agar-Agar: Agar-agar, produced from seaweed, is a vegan substitute for gelatin in recipes like jellies or puddings.

Condiments

- Mayonnaise to Vegan Mayo: Many brands offer vegan mayonnaise made from plant-based oils, great for sandwiches or dressings.
- Worcestershire Sauce to Vegan Alternatives: Traditional Worcestershire sauce includes anchovies; look for a vegan version for the same umami flavor in dressings and marinades.

Implementing these plant-based swaps into your daily meals can significantly add to a healthier diet and lifestyle. Not only are these swaps beneficial for personal health, but they also have a positive effect on the environment. By gradually incorporating more plant-based foods into your diet, you can enjoy a wide range of flavors and textures while nourishing your body in a sustainable way.

Secret#2:

Hydration for Vitality

Water's Role in Your Diet

Water is the most important nutrient for life. It plays a critical role in almost every vital process in the body. Water makes up about 60% of an adult's body weight and is crucial for keeping the balance of body fluids. These fluids are involved in digestion, absorption, circulation, creation of saliva, transportation of nutrients, and control of body temperature.

Detoxification and Digestion:
Water helps in the process of detoxification by helping to flush toxins out of the body through the kidneys. Adequate hydration

ensures that the kidneys work efficiently. In terms of digestion, water helps to dissolve fats and soluble fiber, allowing these components to pass through the bowels more easily. It also helps in avoiding constipation by softening stools and aiding bowel movements.

Weight Management:

Drinking water can help in weight loss and management. Often, the body confuses thirst with hunger. Drinking water before meals can lead to a reduced calorie intake as it provides a sense of fullness. Additionally, hydration can improve metabolism, which plays a significant role in weight management.

Skin Health:

Proper hydration can improve skin health. Dehydration often makes the skin look more dry and wrinkled, which can be improved with proper water. Water helps to replenish skin tissues, moisturize the skin, and improve its elasticity.

Physical Performance:

Hydration is important for maintaining peak physical performance. During intense exercise, the body loses water through sweat. This loss needs to be compensated as even mild dehydration can affect physical performance, lower endurance, and increase fatigue.

Creative Ways to Stay Hydrated Infused Water

One of the easiest ways to enhance your water intake is by infusing it with fruits, vegetables, or herbs. Lemon, cucumber, berries, mint, and ginger can add flavor to water, making it more fun to drink.

Eat Water-Rich Foods:

Incorporate fruits and veggies with high water content into your diet. Watermelon, cucumber, oranges, strawberries, and lemons are some examples. These foods not only help with hydration but also provide important vitamins and minerals.

Set Regular Reminders:

In today's busy lifestyle, it's easy to forget to drink water. Setting notes on your phone or using a hydration tracking app can help you remember to take regular sips throughout the day.

Carry a Reusable Water Bottle:

Having a water bottle on hand at all times pushes you to drink more water. Choose a bottle you enjoy using and make a habit of filling it up several times a day.

Herbal Teas and Flavored Water:

Herbal teas, both hot and cold, can be a hydrating and caffeine-free option to water. Similarly, sparkling or flavored water (without added sugar) can be a more interesting way to hydrate than plain water.

Start and End Your Day with Water:

Make it a habit to drink a glass of water as soon as you wake up and before you go to bed. This ensures that you start and end your day with water.

Track Your Intake:

Keeping track of how much water you drink can be encouraging. There are many ways to do this, from simple tally marks in a notebook to sophisticated apps that log your diet.

Use a Straw:

Some people find that they drink more water when using a straw. This can be especially useful when you're at work or moving.

Drink Water Before, During, and After Meals:

Drinking water before eating can lower appetite, during meals can aid in digestion, and after meals helps to flush out any remaining food particles and aids digestion.

Listen to Your Body:

Learn to spot the signs of dehydration, which can include dry mouth, fatigue, and dark-colored urine. Responding to these signs by drinking water is crucial for keeping hydration.

Hydration is a basic aspect of health and vitality. By adopting these creative and simple strategies, staying hydrated can become an enjoyable and effortless part of your daily routine. Remember, the benefits of hydration stretch far beyond just quenching thirst; they permeate every aspect of health and well-being.

Secret #3

Smart Snacking Habits

Smart snacking is about picking foods that offer both nutritional value and satisfaction. Nutrient-rich snacks provide important vitamins, minerals, fiber, and protein, rather than just empty calories. These nutrients are crucial for keeping energy levels, supporting metabolism, and ensuring overall health.

Mix of Macronutrients:

A good snack should have a mix of macronutrients - carbohydrates, proteins, and healthy fats. This combination helps in stabilizing blood sugar levels and offers a sustained energy source. For instance, mixing a carbohydrate like an apple with a protein such as a handful of nuts can keep you fuller for longer and provide a steady energy release.

Portion Control:

Paying attention to portion amounts is key in smart snacking. Overeating, even healthy snacks, can lead to needless calorie consumption. It's important to be mindful of the amount and to listen to the body's hunger and fullness cues.

Snack Ideas for Energy and Satiety

- Greek Yogurt and Berries: Greek yogurt is rich in protein, while berries provide vitamins and fiber. This snack is satisfying and good for gut health.

- Hummus and Veggies: Hummus, made from beans, is a good source of protein and fiber. Pair it with veggies like carrots, cucumbers, or bell peppers for a crunchy and nutritious snack.

- Nut Butter and Fruit: Apple slices or a banana with a spoonful of almond or peanut butter offer a great mix of sweet and savory, along with a good balance of carbs, protein, and healthy fats.

- Mixed Nuts: Nuts are nutrient-dense, giving healthy fats, proteins, and various vitamins and minerals. A small amount can be a filling and energy-boosting snack.

- Whole Grain Crackers with Cheese: Choose whole grain crackers for fiber and pair them with a bit of cheese for protein and calcium. This combination is satisfying and helps keep energy levels steady.

- Trail Mix: Make your own trail mix with a mixture of nuts, seeds, dried fruit, and whole grain cereals. It's a great on-the-go snack that gives a quick energy boost.

- Popcorn: Air-popped popcorn is a low-calorie, high-fiber snack. Avoid heavy butter and salt; instead, try seasoning with herbs or a sprinkle of nutritional yeast for a cheesy flavor.

- Roasted Chickpeas: These are a crunchy, protein-rich snack. Season them with your favorite spices for a tasty treat.

- Smoothies: Blend together fruits, veggies, and a protein source like Greek yogurt or a scoop of protein powder. Smoothies are a great way to pack in several nutrients in a delicious way.

- Energy Bars: Choose bars with minimal added sugars and a good mix of natural foods like nuts, seeds, and whole grains.

- Cottage Cheese and Pineapple: Cottage cheese is high in protein, and when paired with pineapple, it offers a delightful mix of savory and sweet flavors.

- Avocado Toast: A slice of whole-grain bread topped with avocado offers healthy fats, fiber, and a range of vitamins and minerals. It's both satisfying and healthy.

- Dark Chocolate and Almonds: For a treat, a small amount of dark chocolate with almonds can satisfy sweet cravings while giving antioxidants and healthy fats.

- Edamame: These young soybeans are rich in protein, fiber, and different vitamins and minerals. Lightly salted or seasoned, they make for a delicious and filling snack.

Incorporating these smart eating habits and ideas into your daily routine can make a significant difference in your overall diet. Not only do they provide the necessary energy to get through the day, but they also contribute to a balanced and nutritious diet, making you feel fuller and more satisfied between meals. Remember, the key to smart snacking is to choose nutrient-rich foods and be aware of portion sizes.

Secret #4

Balancing Macronutrients

Understanding Proteins, Carbs, and Fats

Proteins:

Proteins are important for the growth, repair, and maintenance of body tissues. They're made up of amino acids, which are the building blocks for muscles, skin, enzymes, and hormones. High-quality protein sources include lean meats, chicken, fish, dairy products, eggs, legumes, and soy products. For vegetarians and vegans, combining different plant-based protein sources is important to ensure all essential amino acids are consumed.

Carbohydrates:

Starches are the fundamental energy hotspot for the body. They separate into glucose, which drives your cerebrum and muscles. There are two kinds of sugars: straightforward and convoluted. Simple carbs, found in fruits, milk, and sweeteners, are absorbed quickly and provide instant energy. Complex carbs, found in whole grains, legumes, and veggies, take longer to digest and provide sustained energy. They are also high in fiber, which helps in digestion and satiety.

Fats:

Fats are important for energy, supporting cell growth, and protecting organs. They also help the body receive vitamins A, D, E, and K. Fats can be saturated, unsaturated, or trans fats. Unsaturated fats (found in nuts, seeds, fish, and vegetable oils) are considered good for heart health. Saturated fats should be eaten in moderation, and trans fats (found in processed and fried foods) should be avoided as much as possible.

How to Balance Your Plate

Adjusting these macronutrients is critical to a sound eating routine. The possibility of "My Plate" by the USDA can be a useful aide:

- Around 50% of Your Plate - Products of the soil: These ought to cover a portion of your plate. Go for the gold of varieties to guarantee a large number of supplements.

- One-Quarter of Your Plate – Protein: This part of the plate should be filled with protein-rich foods. Plant-based proteins can be especially helpful for health and the environment.

- One-Quarter of Your Plate – Whole Grains: Choose whole carbs like brown rice, quinoa, whole wheat pasta, or bread. These complex carbs provide fiber and important nutrients.

A Small Portion of Healthy Fats:
Include a small amount of healthy fats in each meal. This could be in the form of a drizzle of olive oil, a piece of nuts, or avocado.

- Dairy or Dairy option: Include a serving of dairy or a calcium-fortified dairy option. This could be a glass of milk, a cup of yogurt, or a bit of cheese.

- Portion Control: Be aware of portion sizes. Even healthy foods can add to weight gain if eaten in large quantities.

- Listen to Your Body: Pay attention to your body's hunger and fullness cues. Eating slowly and mindfully can help in spotting these signals.

- Variety is Key: Vary your protein, fat, and carbohydrate sources to ensure a broad range of nutrients. This also keeps dinners interesting and flavorful.

- Hydration: Don't forget about water. Staying well-hydrated is crucial for overall health and can help in digestion and metabolism.

While focused on macronutrients, it's also important to limit the intake of added sugars and heavily processed foods.

Balancing macronutrients is not about tight limitations or complex diet plans. It's about making informed food choices that add to a well-rounded and nutritious diet. By understanding the role of proteins, carbs, and fats, and learning how to balance them

on your plate, you can create meals that are
satisfying, delicious, and healthy.

Secret #5

Mindful Eating Techniques

Mindful eating is about understanding the deep link between our mind and our eating habits. It's not just what we eat, but how, why, and when we eat that counts. This approach recognizes that our eating habits are often driven by emotional factors like stress, boredom, or habit, rather than hunger.

Physical Responses to Food:

Our body's physical response to food is closely tied to our mental state. Stress, for example, can affect digestion and how our body processes food. Being mindful helps in spotting true hunger cues and differentiating them from emotional or stress-related eating.

Mind-Body Harmony:

Mindful eating is about building harmony between mind and body. It encourages a deeper knowledge and appreciation of food, its source, its preparation, and its benefits to our bodies. This awareness leads to a healthier relationship with food, where eating becomes an intentional act rather than an automatic habit.

Strategies for Mindful Eating Eat Without Distractions

1. Avoid eating while watching TV, studying, or using your phone. Distractions can lead to overeating as they prevent you

from paying attention to your body's fullness cues.

2. **Engage All Senses:**

Focus on the smell, taste, surface, and look of your food. This can assist you with partaking in your feasts more and improve the general eating experience.

3. **Bite Gradually and Completely:**

Set aside some margin to appropriately bite your food. This guides in assimilation and gives your body time to perceive when it is full.

4.   Perceive   Yearning   and   Totality Prompts:

Figure out how to detect when you are genuinely ravenous and when you are full. Quit eating when you feel serenely full, not when you are full.

5. Understand Emotional Triggers:

Be aware of emotional causes that lead to eating when not hungry. Find other ways to deal with feelings like stress, anxiety, or boredom.

6. Practice Gratitude for Your Food:

Before eating, take a moment to show gratitude for your meal. This can help create a deeper appreciation for the nourishment you are about to receive.

7. **Eat Regularly and Don't Skip Meals:**

Skipping meals can lead to overeating later. Regular, balanced meals help keep steady blood sugar levels and reduce cravings.

8. **Portion Control:**

Serve yourself smaller amounts and decide if you need more only after you have finished eating what's on your plate.

9. **Mindful Meal Planning:**

Plan meals and drinks ahead of time. This helps in making conscious choices about what to eat, focusing on nutritious and enjoyable options.

10. **Reflect Post-Meal:**

After eating, take a moment to think about how you feel. Did the meal please you?

How has it changed your mood or energy levels?

Mindful eating is a powerful tool for building a healthier relationship with food. It's not about restriction or dieting, but about experiencing food more deeply and with full awareness. By practicing these techniques, you can enjoy meals more, improve digestion, and naturally regulate your eating habits for better general health and well-being.

Secret #6

Sugar Intake Management

Excessive sugar intake can lead to instant effects like energy spikes followed by crashes, impacting mood and productivity. In the long term, it greatly increases the risk of various health issues, including obesity, type 2 diabetes, heart disease, certain cancers, and dental problems.

Role in Chronic Diseases:

High sugar consumption is closely linked with the formation of chronic diseases. It can lead to insulin resistance, a precursor to diabetes, and add to increased inflammation in the body, a risk factor for heart disease and other chronic conditions.

Impact on Mental Health:

Emerging research suggests a link between high sugar diets and mental health disorders, including depression and anxiety. Sugar can affect brain function and mood control, leading to feelings of irritability and fatigue.

Weight Gain and Metabolism:

Sugar, especially added sugars found in processed foods, is a big contributor to obesity. It's high in calories and lacks nutritional value, leading to weight gain. Additionally, it can disrupt the normal functioning of hormones that control hunger and satiety, leading to overeating.

Tips for Reducing Sugar in Your Diet

1. **Read Food Labels:**

Become familiar with reading ingredient labels to spot hidden sugars. Look for terms like sucrose, fructose, dextrose, and high-fructose corn syrup.

2. **Reduce Sugary Beverages:**

Cut back on sodas, energy drinks, and fruit juices with extra sugars. Opt for water, herbal drinks, or infuse water with fruits for taste.

3. **Choose Natural Sweeteners:**

Use honey, maple syrup, or agave juice in moderation instead of white sugar. These natural sweeteners contain more nutrients and are often sweeter, so you can use less.

4. Eat Whole Fruits Instead of Processed Snacks:

Replace sugary snacks with whole fruits. The natural sugars in vegetables are less concentrated and come with fiber, vitamins, and minerals.

5. Avoid Processed and Packaged Foods:

Processed foods often contain a shocking amount of added sugars. Opt for whole, raw foods as much as possible.

6. Beware of Low-fat and "Diet" Foods:

These goods often contain added sugars to improve taste. Always check the chemical list and nutrition facts.

7. **Cook and Bake at Home:**

Preparing meals and snacks at home helps you to control the amount and type of sweeteners used.

8. **Reduce Sugar Gradually:**

Continuously reduce how much sugar you add to food sources and beverages. Your taste buds will change over the long run.

9. **Spice it Up:**

Use spices like cinnamon, nutmeg, and vanilla to add sweetness to foods without sugar.

10. **Limit Desserts and Treats:**

Save sugary desserts for special events. Explore healthier dessert ideas that use less sugar or natural sweeteners.

11. **Focus on Overall Diet Quality:**
Incorporate a balanced diet rich in veggies, fruits, whole grains, lean proteins, and healthy fats. A well-rounded diet can lessen cravings for sugary foods.

Managing sugar intake is important for maintaining good health and preventing chronic diseases. By being mindful of sugar consumption and making gradual changes, you can greatly improve your diet and overall well-being. Remember, reducing sugar is not about deprivation but about making better choices that can lead to a more balanced and nutritious lifestyle.

Secret #7

The Importance of Breakfast Kickstarting Your Metabolism

Metabolic Boost:

Eating breakfast can jumpstart your metabolism, telling your body to start burning calories for the day. After a night of fasting, a nutritious breakfast provides the energy your body needs to begin working optimally. Skipping breakfast can lead to a slower metabolism as the body tries to retain energy.

Balanced Blood Sugar Levels:

A morning meal helps to balance blood sugar levels, which is crucial for controlling appetite and energy levels throughout the day. Consistent blood sugar levels avoid energy crashes and can help curb overeating later in the day.

Enhanced Cognitive Function:

Breakfast also plays a major role in improving focus and concentration. Studies have shown that eating a nutritious breakfast can improve memory, attention, and the speed of processing information.

Quick and Healthy Breakfast Ideas Overnight Oats:

Combine rolled oats with yogurt or milk, chia seeds, and your favorite fruits. Leave it in the fridge overnight for a quick and nutritious grab-and-go choice in the morning.

Greek Yogurt with Nuts and Berries:

Greek yogurt is high in protein and low in sugar.Top it with berries for vitamins and nuts for healthy fats and an extra protein boost.

Smoothie Bowls:

Blend fruits, greens, and a protein source like Greek yogurt or a scoop of protein powder. Top with seeds, nuts, and fresh fruit.

Whole Grain Toast with Avocado and Egg:

A slice of whole-grain bread topped with smashed avocado and a poached or scrambled egg offers a balance of healthy fats, protein, and fiber.

Banana and Nut Butter Toast:

For an easy yet filling breakfast, spread almond or peanut butter on whole-grain toast and top with banana slices. This offers a good mix of complex carbs, healthy fats, and protein.

Vegetable Omelette or Scramble:

Whisk together eggs and cook with a mix of your favorite veggies like spinach, tomatoes, and bell peppers. Add some cheese or avocado for extra taste and nutrients.

Protein Pancakes:

Make pancakes using oat flour, protein powder, and egg. Serve with fresh fruit or a drop of honey for sweetness.

Cottage Cheese with Pineapple or Peaches:

Cottage cheese is a great source of protein. Pair it with fruit like pineapple or peaches for a sweet and filling breakfast.

Breakfast Burrito:

Fill a whole-wheat tortilla with cooked eggs, beans, cheese, and salsa. You can make these in advance and freeze them for a quick, microwaveable breakfast choice.

Quinoa Fruit Salad:

Mix cooked rice with diced fruits, a splash of lemon juice, and a drizzle of honey. Quinoa is a great source of plant-based energy and fiber.

Whole Grain Cereal with Milk or Plant-Based Milk:

Choose a high-fiber, low-sugar cereal and serve it with milk or a plant-based milk substitute. Top with fruits for extra nutrients. Incorporating these quick and healthy breakfast ideas can greatly improve your morning routine. A nutritious breakfast not only kick-starts your metabolism but also sets the tone for the rest of the day, helping you make healthier choices and keep your energy levels. Remember, the key to a helpful breakfast is balance – include a good mix of protein, healthy fats, and complex carbohydrates.

Secret #8

Meal Prepping for Success

Meal prepping includes planning and preparing meals ahead of time. It's an effective strategy for keeping a healthy diet, especially for those with busy lifestyles. By dedicating a few hours to meal prep, you can ensure that you have healthy, balanced meals throughout the week, reducing the desire to opt for fast food or processed snacks.

Time and Cost Efficiency:
Meal prepping saves time during the week and can also be cost-effective. Buying ingredients in bulk and preparing meals at home can reduce food waste and lower total

food expenses. It also reduces the time spent cooking and cleaning up during the week.

Meal Prep Tips and Tricks

Start with a Plan:

Before you shop, decide what you'll eat for breakfast, lunch, dinner, and snacks. Make a grocery list to avoid buying unnecessary things.

Choose Versatile Ingredients:

Opt for items that can be used in multiple meals. For example, cook a big batch of quinoa or brown rice to use in salads, stir-fries, and as a side dish.

Invest in Quality Containers:

Use good quality, microwave-safe, and freezer-friendly packages. Portioning food into individual containers can make it easy to grab and go.

Batch Cook and Freeze:

Prepare large batches of meals that freeze well, like soups, stews, and casseroles. Freeze in pieces for easy defrosting and reheating.

Prep Ingredients, Not Just Meals:

If you prefer more variety, prep items instead of full meals. Cook proteins, chop vegetables, and make sauces to mix and match for different meals.

Keep It Simple:

Don't over complicate your meal prep. Simple recipes with fewer items can be just as nutritious and less time-consuming.

Incorporate Raw Foods:

Include fresh fruits and raw veggies for snacks or to add to meals. They require no cooking and add important nutrients and fiber to your diet.

Utilize Crock Pots or Instant Pots:

Slow cookers and instant pots are great for easy, one-pot meals. They can cook big quantities with minimal effort.

Season Differently:

If you're cooking a big batch of a single ingredient, season portions differently to add variety throughout the week.

Schedule a Prep Day:

Dedicate a specific day and time each week for meal prep. This regularity helps in making meal prepping a habit.

Keep Snacks Handy:

Prepare healthy snacks like chopped veggies, fruits, nuts, or yogurt to curb hunger between meals.

Label Your Meals:

Labeling meals with dates and ingredients can help keep track of what you have and ensure food safety.

Meal prepping is an effective way to keep a healthy diet and simplify your weekly routine. It takes the guesswork out of what to eat, helps control portion sizes, and ensures that you have nutritious options easily available. By incorporating these meal prep tips and tricks, you can make healthy eating a useful and enjoyable part of your life.

Secret #9

Incorporating Superfoods

What Are Superfoods?

The word "superfoods" refers to foods that are highly nutrient-dense, meaning they are packed with vitamins, minerals, antioxidants, and other health-promoting properties. Unlike other healthy foods, superfoods are known for their high concentration of essential nutrients and their associated benefits, which can include better health, energy, and disease prevention. It's important to note that "superfood" is not a scientific term but rather a marketing word that has gained popularity.

Characteristics of Superfoods

Rich in Nutrients: Superfoods offer a high density of nutrients compared to their caloric content.

Antioxidant Properties: Many superfoods contain antioxidants, which help combat oxidative stress and reduce the chance of chronic diseases.

Fiber Content: Superfoods often have high fiber content, beneficial for digestion and keeping a healthy gut.

Minimally Processed: Superfoods are usually whole, natural foods that have undergone minimal processing.

Examples of Superfoods

Berries: Such as blueberries, strawberries, and raspberries, known for their high amounts of antioxidants.

Leafy Greens: Like spinach, kale, and Swiss chard, packed with vitamins A, C, and K, as well as fiber, iron, and calcium.

Nuts and Seeds: Including almonds, flaxseeds, and chia seeds, which provide healthy fats, protein, and different micronutrients.

Ancient Grains: Quinoa, amaranth, and buckwheat, giving a high protein content and rich in fiber.

Green Tea: Known for its antioxidant qualities and beneficial effects on metabolism.

Avocado: High in healthy monounsaturated fats, fiber, and several important vitamins and minerals.

Dark Chocolate: Rich in vitamins, iron, magnesium, and fiber.

Legumes: Such as lentils and beans, which are high in protein, fiber, and complex carbohydrates.

Fatty Fish: Like salmon and tuna, sources of Omega-3 fatty acids.

Cruciferous Vegetables: Broccoli, Brussels sprouts, and cauliflower, known for their cancer-fighting qualities.

Simple Methods for remembering Superfoods for Your Eating routine

Integrating superfoods into your eating routine doesn't need to be troublesome or costly. Here are a simple methods for adding them into ordinary dinners:

Begin with Breakfast:

Add berries to your yogurt, oatmeal, or cereal.

Make shakes with spinach, kale, or avocado.

Use chia or flax seeds as a topping for toast or in drinks.

Snack Smart:

Snack on nuts like almonds or walnuts.

Choose foods like apples or bananas.

Enjoy dark chocolate in moderation.

Super Salads:

Create salads with a base of fresh greens like spinach or kale.

Add a range of colorful vegetables, nuts, seeds, and a portion of grilled salmon or chicken.

Power-Packed Main Courses:

Use quinoa or amaranth as a side item or in place of rice.

Incorporate legumes into soups, stews, or as a meat substitute in meals like tacos or burgers.

Add cruciferous veggies to stir-fries, casseroles, and pasta dishes.

Healthy Drinks:

Replace coffee with green tea.

Make fresh fruit or veggie juices, combining items like kale, carrots, and apples.

Dressings and Sauces:

Use avocado or nuts to make creamy dressings and sauces.

Include garlic and turmeric, known for their anti-inflammatory qualities, in your recipes.

Desserts and Baking:

Bake with almond or coconut flour.

Use dark chocolate chips in baked cookies or muffins.

Create desserts based around fruits, like a berry parfait.

Experiment with International Cuisine: Many international dishes easily incorporate superfoods. For example, Indian curries often use turmeric and lentils, while Japanese food includes seaweed and green tea.

Meal Prep with Superfoods

When meal prepping, include at least one vegetable in each meal. For example, prepare a batch of quinoa at the start of the week to use in different dishes.

Mindful Additions:

Find small ways to add superfoods to your current favorite meals, like adding spinach to a pizza or berries to pancakes.

Educate Yourself:

Stay updated about new superfoods and their benefits. However, always ensure that any new food fits into your dietary wants and restrictions.

Balance and Moderation:

Remember that while superfoods are helpful, they should be part of a balanced diet. No single food can give every one of the fundamental supplements.

Incorporating superfoods into your diet can be an enjoyable and beneficial effort. These nutrient-rich foods can enhance the quality of your diet and may help to better health and well-being. The key is variety and moderation, ensuring that your food is balanced and diverse.

Secret #10

Consistency Over Perfection

The pursuit of a healthy lifestyle is often marred by the drive for perfection – a flawless diet, an unbreakable exercise routine, and unwavering willpower. However, the key to long-term success in health and wellness comes not in perfection, but in consistency. Embracing imperfection means admitting that setbacks are a normal part of any journey and that progress, no matter how small, is still progress.

Sustainable Habits:

Consistency is about building sustainable habits over time. It includes making healthier choices more often than not, but also allowing room for flexibility and enjoyment. This approach reduces the pressure and guilt often linked with strict diets or rigorous fitness regimes, making it more likely to stick with healthy habits in the long run.

Long-Term Mindset:
Adopting a long-term mindset is important. Health and wellness are not achieved quickly or through short-term diets; they are the result of ongoing, consistent efforts. A long-term perspective helps in making decisions that are not just beneficial now, but also conducive to future well-being.

How to Stay Motivated and On Track Set Realistic Goals

Establish achievable goals that inspire you. Unrealistic or vague goals can lead to frustration and loss of drive. Separate major objectives into more modest, sensible advances.

Make a Daily schedule:

A routine gives requests and makes it simpler to remain reliable. Set explicit times for dinners, work out, and other health undertakings. Over the long run, these will become typical pieces of your day.

Keep tabs on Your Development:

Keep a log or use applications to keep tabs on your development. Celebrate little wins and ponder what you've gained from any mishaps.

Track down Pleasant Exercises:

Pick kinds of activity and quality food varieties that you really appreciate. You're bound to be consistent on the off chance that you're having a good time and not simply making a halfhearted effort.

Show restraint toward Yourself:

Comprehending that change requires some investment. Be patient and kind to yourself, particularly on days when things don't go as expected.

Fabricate an Emotionally supportive network:

Encircle yourself with individuals who support and rouse you. Friends, family, or online communities can offer encouragement, help, and a feeling of accountability.

Learn from Setbacks:

Instead of dwelling on setbacks, view them as learning chances. Analyze what led to the loss and how you can handle it differently in the future.

Stay Flexible:

Life is uncertain, and rigid plans may not always work. Be open to adjusting your goals and tactics as needed.

Focus on Health, Not Just Appearance:
Shift your attention from solely aesthetic goals to overall health and well-being. This perspective encourages a more holistic and sustainable strategy.

Practice Mindfulness:
Be present and mindful in your daily tasks, whether it's eating, exercising, or resting. Mindfulness helps in making intentional choices and appreciating the path.

Reward Yourself:
Celebrate your success with non-food rewards, like a new book, a relaxing bath, or time for a favorite hobby.

Visualize Success:

Use visualization techniques to imagine reaching your goals. This can improve your confidence and motivation.

Educate Yourself:

Knowledge is power. The more you understand about nutrition, exercise, and wellness, the better equipped you are to make informed choices.

Avoid the All-or-Nothing Mindset:

Don't let one slip-up derail your entire effort. Accept that flaws are part of the process and move on.

Prioritize Self-Care:

Ensure you're getting enough sleep, handling stress, and taking time for yourself. Self-care is integral to keeping motivation and overall well-being.

Remain Adaptable:

Be ready to adapt your strategy to new situations, whether it's a change in schedule, lifestyle, or goals.

Stay Inspired:

Find sources of inspiration, whether it's through motivational books, podcasts, or following health and wellness influencers who connect with your journey.

Reflect Regularly:

Take time to reflect on your trip, the changes you've experienced, and what you've learned about yourself.

Focus on Non-Scale Victories:

Acknowledge and celebrate improvements in your energy levels, mood, strength, and other non-scale wins.

Revisit and Revise Goals:

Regularly revisit your goals to ensure they still fit with your values and lifestyle. Adjust them as needed to keep them current and motivating.

Consistency over perfection in health and fitness is about making incremental changes and sticking to them over time. It's a journey of self-discovery and growth, where the end goal is not a perfect state, but a healthier, happier, and more balanced life. Remember, it's not about being flawless; it's about being consistent and resilient, and always trying to be your best self.

Conclusion

Your Journey to a Healthier Year

As we wrap up the study of the "Top 10 Diet Secrets for a Vibrant New Year," it's clear that starting on a journey to a healthier year is not just about the foods we eat, but also about our overall approach to health and wellness. Each secret offers a piece to the puzzle of creating a sustainable, balanced, and fulfilling lifestyle.

Summing Up the Diet Secrets

Power of Plant-Based Choices:
Emphasizing plant-based foods for their various health benefits and how simple swaps can enrich your diet.

Hydration for Vitality:

Understanding the crucial role of water in overall health and adopting creative ways to stay hydrated.

Smart Snacking Habits:

Choosing nutrient-rich snacks for energy and satiety to support a balanced diet and avoid overeating.

Balancing Macronutrients:

The value of a balanced intake of proteins, carbs, and fats for optimal health and how to achieve this balance in your meals.

Mindful Eating Techniques:

The connection between mind and body in eating habits and strategies for building a more mindful relationship with food.

Sugar Intake Management:

Recognizing the effect of sugar on health and practical tips for reducing sugar consumption in your diet.

The Importance of Breakfast:

How a healthy breakfast kick starts metabolism and ideas for quick, nutritious breakfast choices.

Meal Prepping for Success:

The benefits of planning and preparing meals ahead for healthy eating and tips to make meal prepping effective and fun.

Incorporating Superfoods:

Understanding what superfoods are and easy ways to include them in your diet for an extra health boost.

Consistency Over Perfection:

Emphasizing the importance of consistent efforts over aiming for perfection for long-term success in health and wellness.

Encouraging Sustainable Lifestyle Changes
As you step into the new year, remember that these tips are not just short-term fixes but are meant to inspire long-lasting changes. Health is a journey, not a goal, and it's about making small, sustainable changes that add up over time. Here are some final thoughts to support you on this journey:

Personalize Your Approach:

Adapt these secrets to fit your unique lifestyle, tastes, and goals. What works for one individual may not work for another, and that is not a problem.

Progress, Not Perfection:

Focus on making progress, however small it may be. Every healthy choice is a step in the right way.

Be Patient and Kind to Yourself:

Change takes time, and there will be difficulties. Treat yourself with care and patience.

Seek Support and Community:

Share your story with others. Whether it's friends, family, or an online group, having support can make a significant difference.

Celebrate Your Achievements:

Take time to notice and celebrate your achievements, no matter how small they may seem.

Stay Flexible and Open to Learning:

Be open to trying new things and adjusting your method as you learn what works best for you.

Prioritize Joy and Enjoyment:

Find joy in the process. Whether it's experimenting with new recipes or finding physical things you love, enjoyment is key to sustainability.

As you move forward, keep these diet hints and tips in mind. They're meant not just to improve your physical health, but to enhance your overall well-being, bringing more energy, vitality, and joy into your life. Here's to a healthier, happy you in the new year!